The Grandparent's G

MW01066040

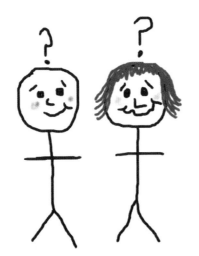

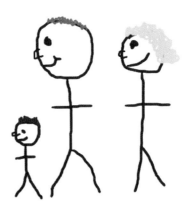

To The Well-Oiled Kid

Written by Mom (Dr. Melissa Shelton)
With help from Ramie Shelton
Illustrated by Melissa, Ramie, & Reiker Shelton

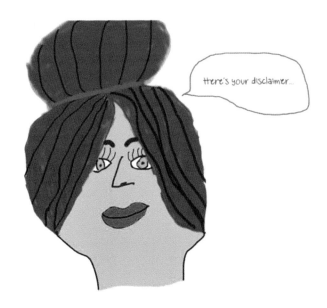

The information in this book is not intended to replace good old fashioned medical care - and is intended for educational purposes only. The author(s) and contributor(s) will assume no liability for any loss or damage of any nature, by the use of any information contained within this publication. If you or a loved one have a health concern, please seek the advice of a qualified health care professional.

When our parents first started to use Essential Oils instead of "over-the-counter" medicines - some of our family members thought we were a bit strange...

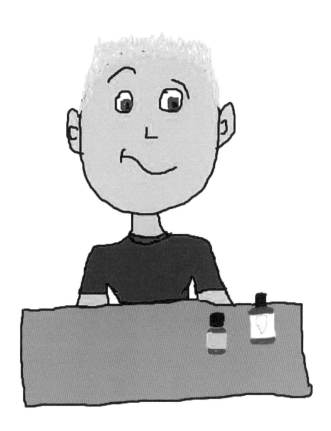

And...

SMELLY!

As time went on – our family members saw some good things in what we were doing...

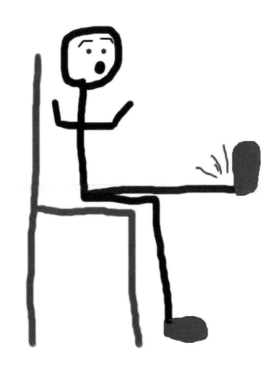

(Grandpa even wanted essential oils applied to his sprained ankle!)

This book is dedicated to all of the reluctant grandparents – trying to "humor" their "stinky" kids' wishes...

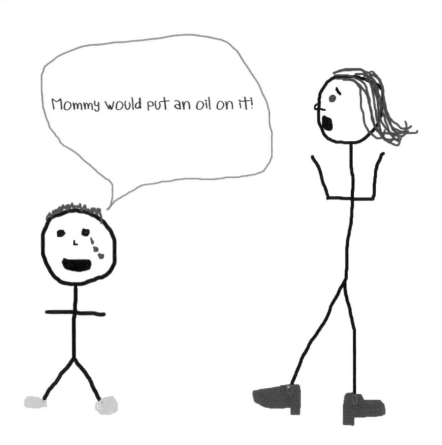

By using Essential Oils on their grandkids...

Here is Mom's list of Essential Oils that she likes our Grandparents to have...

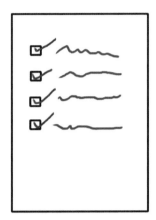

Most of them are in Young Living's Everyday Oils Kit.

Lemon   Valor
Peppermint   Thieves
Lavender   PanAway
Frankincense   Purification

And my mom's favorite – Peace & Calming.

There are a few other oils we like too... (And mom says you get "bonus points" if more than 15 oils are sent along with your grandkids!)

DiGize Essential Oil Blend
Helichrysum Essential Oil
And V-6 Vegetable Oil Complex

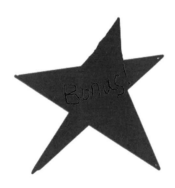

Bonus!

Almost everything can be done with the Everyday Oils Kit though.

Here are the most common "kid" situations and how to use essential oils for them...

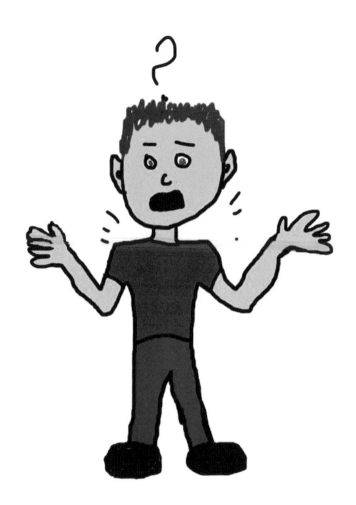

Even when you feel like you don't know WHAT you are doing!

First - you need to have a quick lesson on safety...

#1

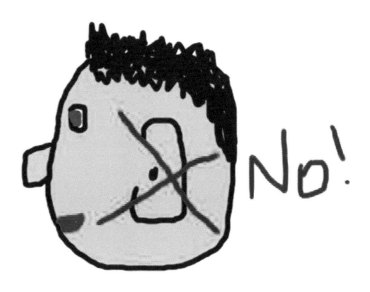

Don't dump oils into an ear...

Don't get essential oils into your eyes. (Note: kids are great at wiping their eyes with oils on their hands!)

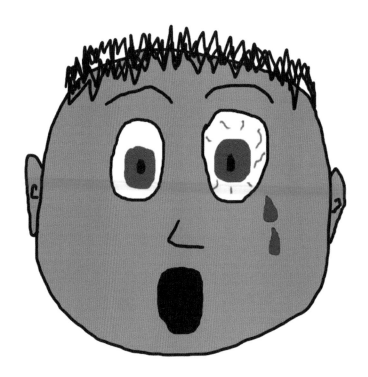

This WILL sting!

When #2 Happens...
(Sorry but because we are kids - and because we are on "your watch" - this WILL happen!)

Never rinse the essential oil away with water. Because water and oil don't mix - it will spread the oils and make things worse. Instead... flush the eye (or any skin that is uncomfortable) with a "Carrier Oil."

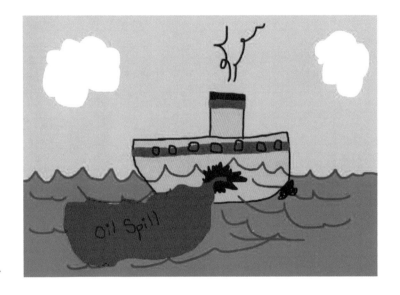

A Carrier Oil is any sort of "fatty" oil - like Olive Oil, Coconut Oil, or Young Living's V-6 Vegetable Oil Complex. But, in an emergency - even butter or a creamer from a restaurant can work.

#4

When in doubt - the safest place to apply essential oils to kids is on the bottom of their feet...

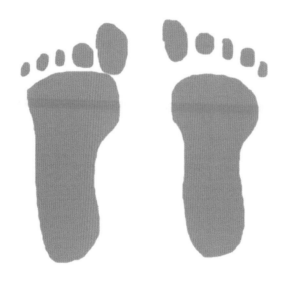

(But, beware... my brother's feet really stink! So it may not be the safest for YOU!)

#5

If at any time there is discomfort on the skin – just apply more carrier oil to the site.

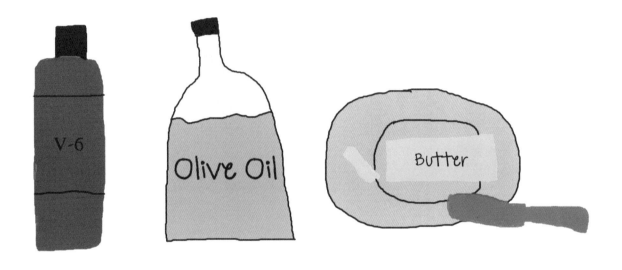

Anything red, cold, hot, or uncomfortable...

#6

Lemon Essential Oil and other citrus oils (like Orange, Tangerine, Bergamot, Lime...) are what my mom calls "photosensitive"... This means that if they are on our skin, and we go out in the sun - we will turn a really weird gray-brown sort of color... (The blend Peace & Calming also has citrus oils in it.)

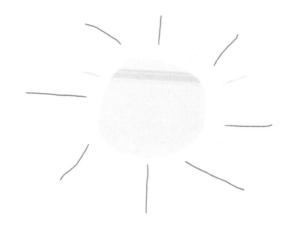

But the funniest thing is that we get to tell you to "stick it where the sun don't shine" - or not to apply a citrus oil to a spot that will be in the sun for about 12-24 hours after application.

Now... Let's go through all of the mischief your grandkids can throw at you!

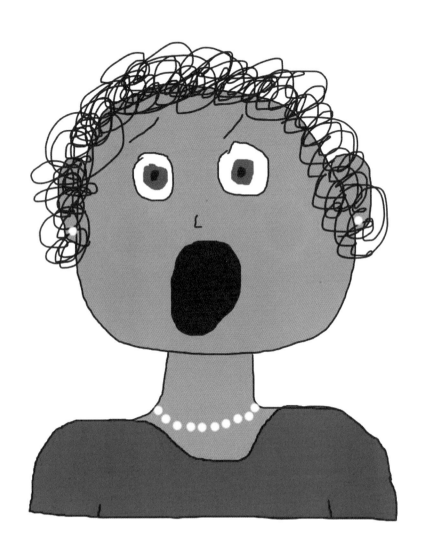

"Grandma... I got gum in my hair!"

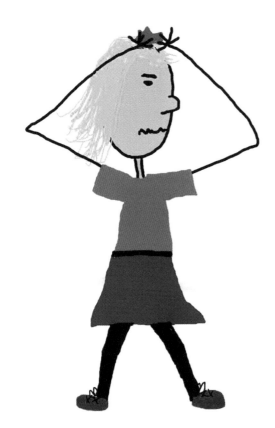

Lemon Oil to the rescue!

Dilute the Lemon Essential Oil 1/2 and 1/2 with the V-6 carrier oil. Apply to the gum and pull out of the hair. The Lemon Oil will make the gum just come right out! Follow with a good shampooing - and NO fancy haircut is needed!

"Look Grandpa! I decorated your windows!"

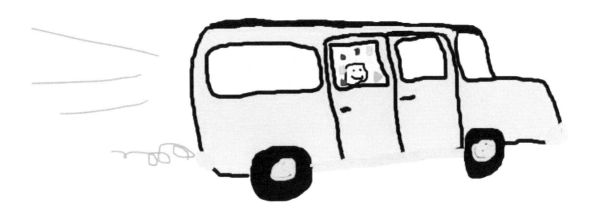

Stickers and sticky things on windows, walls, tables and other places will come off easy with Lemon Oil (just like the gum.)

Just make sure that you test out the Lemon Oil on whatever we stuck things to first - to make sure the essential oil doesn't ruin it. Most of the time - our mom can use the Lemon Oil straight onto the window or sticker without the carrier oil. (She calls this using the oil "neat." We think it is pretty neat too!)

While we are talking about Lemon Oil - it is good to know that it works great for tree sap, pine tar, black top, and other sticky, nasty substances that we can find!

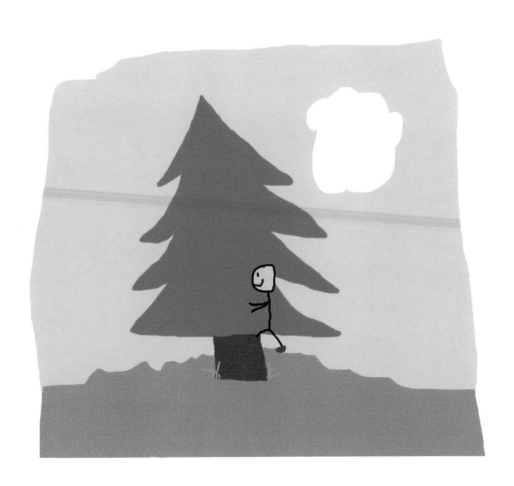

"I don't feel so..."

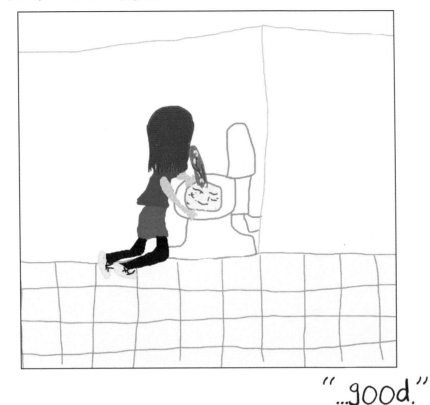

"...good."

Tummy aches are bound to happen - because likely if your kids have essential oils they want you to use - they also have some weird "dietary rules" too!

Pssst...

Between you and me... we know you're gonna give the kids things they are not supposed to have. After all, you raised kids – and they turned out "just fine!"

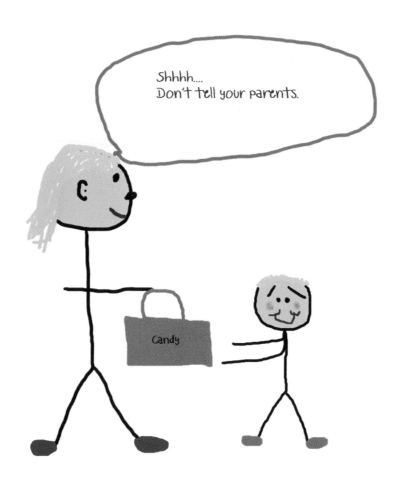

Peppermint Essential Oil or DiGize Essential Oil Blend - can work wonders for those tummy aches!

Place one drop in the belly button...

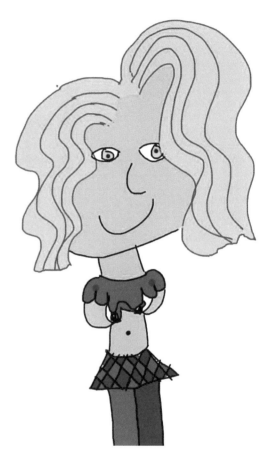

Repeat as needed. (Apply V-6 carrier oil if we complain that it is too cold, too hot, uncomfortable, or if skin gets red.)

"I played in the sun ALL DAY!"

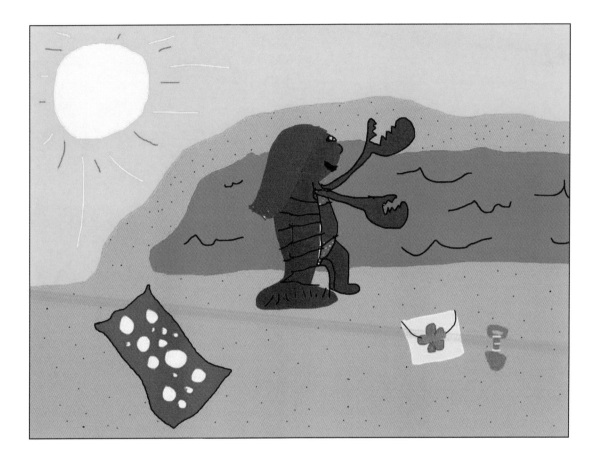

Sunburns will heal faster with Lavender Essential
Oil applied! You can dilute it or apply it neat to
burns. Frankincense, Peppermint, and PanAway
are also good choices.

"It's not THAT cold!"

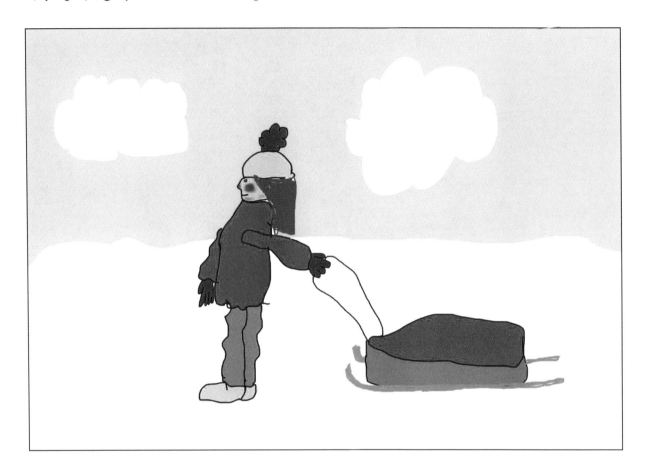

Lavender works on Frostbite too!

"But... We're not tired!"

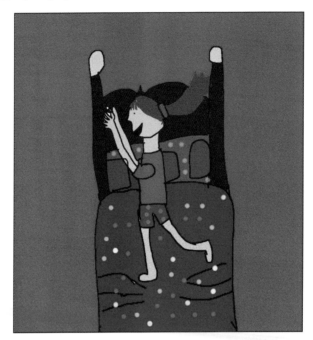

Peace & Calming or Lavender Essential Oil can be applied to the bottom of our feet, rubbed onto our blankets or stuffed animals, misted or diffused into the air...
and...
makes...
us...
tired...

"I miss mommy..."

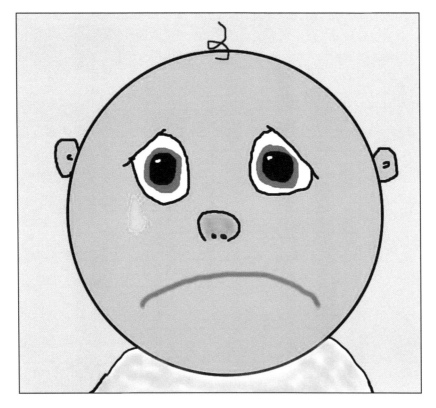

Valor and Peace & Calming Essential Oil Blends are great for making us feel better. You can put them on our feet, in our belly button, or just have us smell them. (If you wear them, we'll smell them when we snuggle...plus you'll smell like mommy and daddy.)

"I helped Grandpa!"

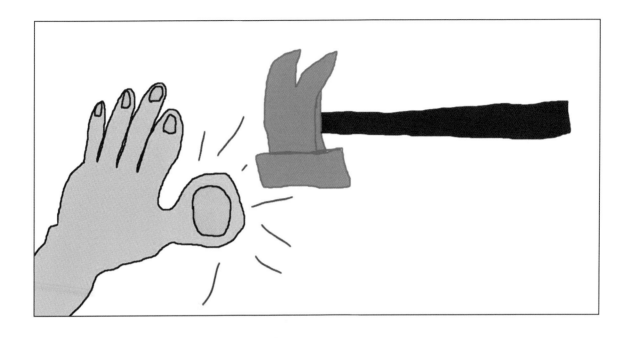

Bumps, bruises, sprained ankles, hammered thumbs, goose eggs... All do great with Valor, Frankincense, Lavender, or PanAway. (Just be careful with PanAway near eyes and delicate tissues - it is minty and can sting a little.)

Usually mom will just apply some of these oils with her finger, right onto the owie - neat or diluted.

Skinned knees and cuts...

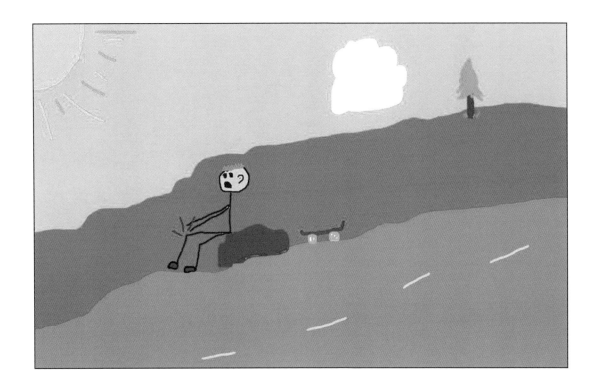

PanAway, Lavender, and Thieves can be used on
these. Any essential oil can sting in an open
wound, but PanAway and Thieves may more than
others. Be ready to dilute it if we complain.
(When I fell out of a tree, I thought it was going to hurt really
bad to put Thieves on my cut - but it DIDN'T!)

If you got those nerdy bonus points - 'cause your kids have WAY too many oils - Helichrysum is awesome for cuts, scrapes, scratches, and bruises.

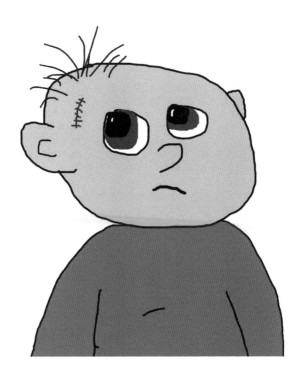

If you have to take us somewhere for stitches... mom says put some Helichrysum on it while you are going to the ER. (Yep, you guessed it, my mom knows this from experience... and it really helped!)

"Let's have a snack!"
"Not before you wash your hands..."

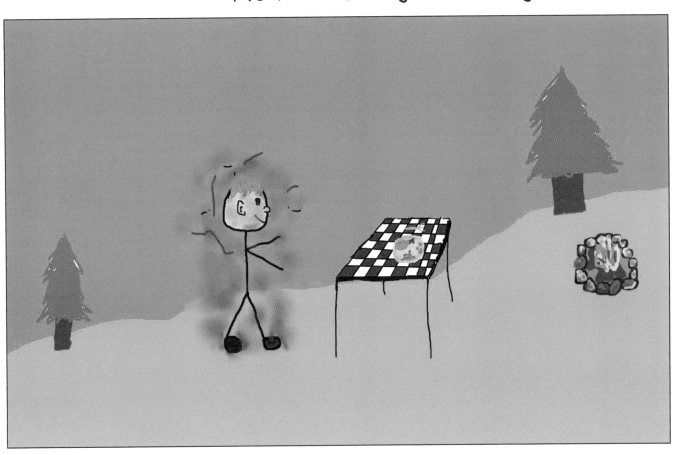

A drop or two of Thieves, Lemon, or Purification Essential Oil rubbed around in our hands can disinfect them.

"Is that a hummingbird or a mosquito?"

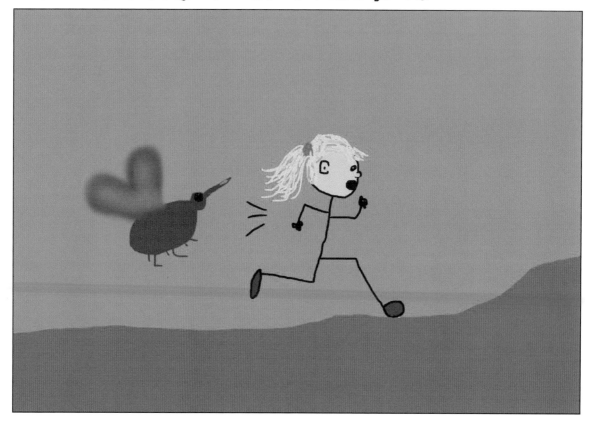

Bee stings, gnat bites, mosquito bites, spider bites...

Purification Essential Oil Blend can repel insects and is good to put on bites to stop the itching or swelling. Mom usually puts it on neat.

"I have a headache..."

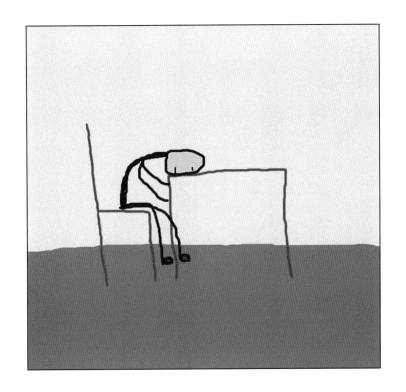

Peppermint, PanAway, Lavender - on the back of the neck, on the feet, or in the belly button can really help. Sometimes Lavender on our temples, or even a drop of Peppermint in our water is extra helpful (shake up the water really good.)

Stuffy noses, coughs, and colds...

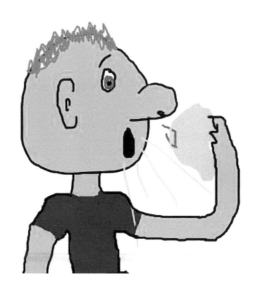

Diffuse Purification, Peppermint, or Thieves in one of those cool mist diffusers or have us smell them from our hands.

Peppermint can be rubbed on our chest - and so can Lemon and Frankincense.

Thieves is great on the bottom of our feet, too!

Sore throats and coughs...

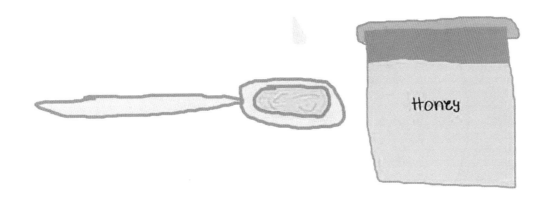

In a teaspoon of Honey or Agave syrup - you can put a drop of Lemon, Peppermint, or Thieves Essential Oil. (Sometimes we put one or two oils.) Mom tells us to hold the honey in our mouth for a while, and let it touch the ouchie part of our throat before we swallow it. The Thieves really helps a bad sore throat, 'cause the Clove Oil in it can numb stuff.

Ear aches...

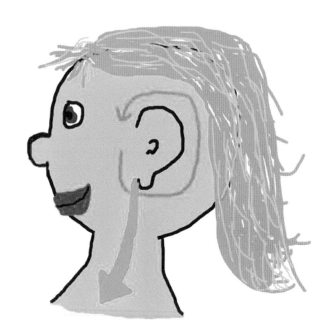

Purification is great when you rub it around the ear, then massage down the Eustachian tube (not the YouTube...)

Just dip your finger into the oil, then massage around the ear. Dip your finger in the oil again, and "milk" down the neck to help drain "gunk" down the Eustachian tube... (Yeah, my mom actually understands this stuff...)

Teething...

Your kid will let you know if this may be needed for your grandkid...

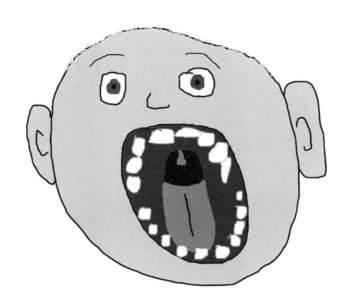

Thieves rubbed onto the gum area (usually diluted 1/2 and 1/2 in coconut oil, olive oil, or V-6) can really numb painful teething. Clove oil can be used too - and is in the Thieves blend of oil.

Growing pains, cramps, and other kid owies...

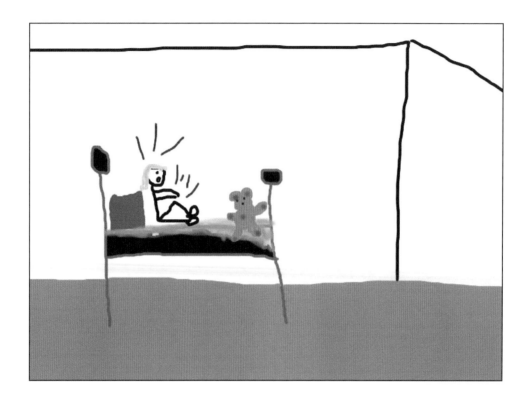

Lavender, Peace & Calming, and PanAway can help sore muscles and aches and pains go away! Just rub them diluted or neat onto the area that needs help.

Shyness and meeting other kids...

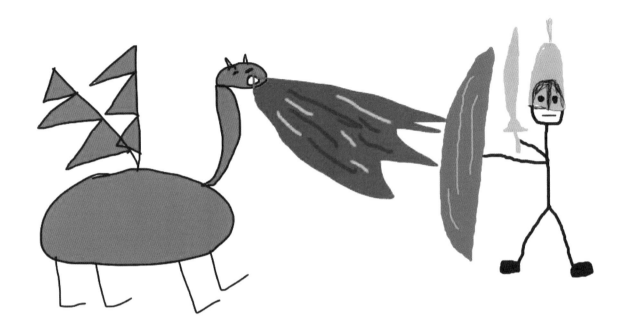

Put a drop or two of Valor onto wrists. Rub
them together, and have the child take a few
deep breaths while holding their wrists together
(veins to veins). This will usually relax us quite a
bit.

(Okay, this one is for my brother...)

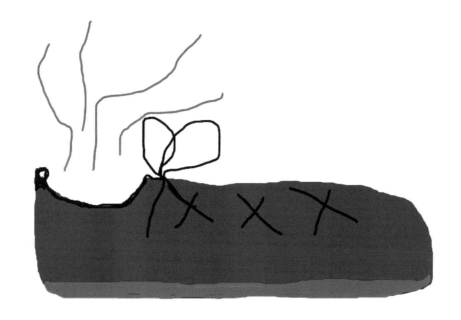

The Sneaker that DIED Inside!

Drip Purification or Thieves right into the shoe and onto the bottom of the ultra-stinky feet!

(And, this one is for Grandma...)

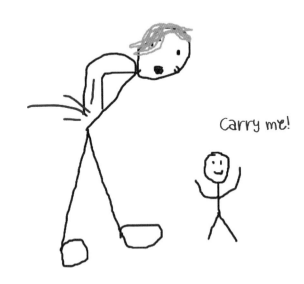

Carry me!

Chronic Carry Me Syndrome

Let's face it - you're bound to try out some of this "new-aged" stuff eventually...

Valor, PanAway, Peppermint, and Lavender are all great on your backache after playing with us kids all weekend!

In this part of the book – we thought it would be good for you to know more about each oil.

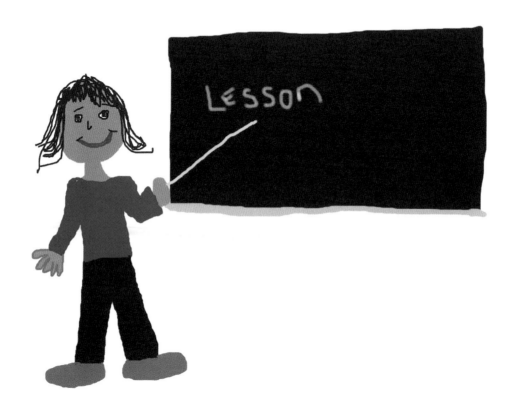

You can skip to the "good stuff" back here if you get bored – or need to know what a particular oil is good for.

Frankincense Essential Oil:

My mom likes to say, "If it's good enough for Baby Jesus... blah, blah, blah..." I think this is her way of saying that Frankincense is a pretty awesome oil, and that we should use it more often.

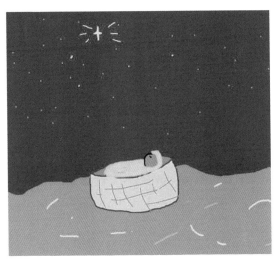

We know it is really good for calming and focusing, but also for cuts, scrapes, bruises, sunburns, skin irritations, headaches, seizures, and concussions. Churches use Frankincense a lot too - and it is used in many kinds of prayers and religions.

Lavender Essential Oil

Good for calming, leg cramps, growing pains, sleeping, bruises, cuts and scrapes, burns, sunburn, frost bite, skin irritations, styes, pink eye, eye infections, headaches, muscle aches, allergies, hives, ringworm... Need we say more?

Basically, this is the all-around perfect oil. It is pretty mild to use, but is strongly antibacterial, antifungal, antiviral - you name it - it does it!

Lemon Essential Oil:

Good for gum, stickers, coughs, sore throats, putting in hot honey water, disinfecting hands, Plantars Warts, flavoring water, fresh smells, antiviral, and antibacterial...

But remember - Lemon is Photosensitive...

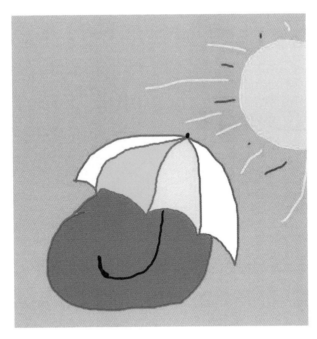

So, stick it where the sun don't shine!

PanAway Essential Oil Blend:

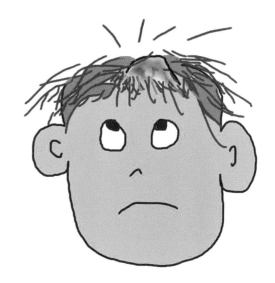

Good for aches, pains, scratches, cuts, scrapes, goose eggs, bruises, sprained ankles, achey grandparents, and headaches.

If you haven't earned the "bonus points" – this blend contains Helichrysum – so is a good "almost bonus points" oil!

PanAway has Wintergreen in it – which can be strong smelling, cold, or irritate eyes or other delicate tissues. You may want to dilute it, or apply to the bottom of feet.

Peace & Calming Essential Oil Blend:

Is good for worried and anxious kids, leg cramps, growing pains, when you can't sleep (or want to jump on the bed instead), helps decrease fighting with siblings - anything that needs peace and calming!

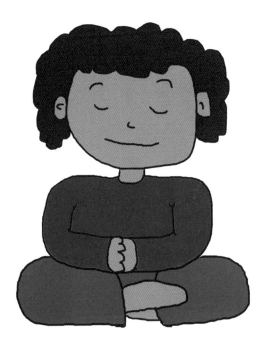

WARNING: Some kids did not read this book and may not experience "Peace and Calming" - and may have MORE get up and go! If this is your grandkid - then use Lavender.

Peppermint Essential Oil:

Good for headaches, upset tummy, clogged nose, congestion, inflammation and pain, coughs, to flavor cookies, cakes, and CANDY, when you are over-heated, sunburn, car sickness, and for perking up tired grandparents.

Remember - Lot's of menthol in Peppermint can mean it feels...

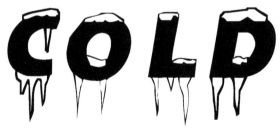

It can also make your eyes tear up, and the strong scent may need to be avoided in very small children.

Purification Essential Oil Blend:

Good for bug bites, spider bites, hives, insect repellant, odor elimination, cuts, scrapes, lacerations (that's the big word my mom uses), diffuse for coughs and colds, rub around ears for ear aches.

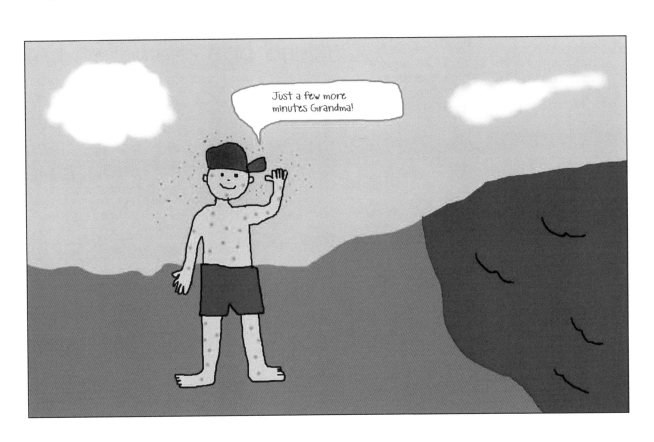

Thieves Essential Oil Blend:

This one is really good for the bottom of the feet or in a diffuser - 'cause it is a little "hot."

Thieves is good for warts, coughs, colds, flu, sore throats, stinky feet and shoes, to disinfect hands, for tooth pain, for teething pain, and is GREAT in hot apple cider (served with gluten free cookies - of course.)

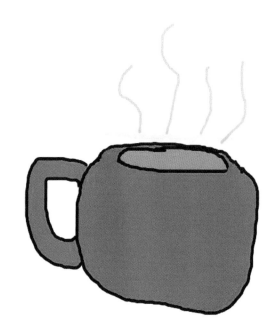

Valor Essential Oil Blend:

Valor means "brave" – so it is great for anytime
we need to have more bravery. It is also really
good for backaches, and lots of people call it
"Chiropractor in a bottle." It's great for lots of
things like shyness, missing our parents,
headaches, motion sickness, to help us fall asleep,
and on bumps and bruises...

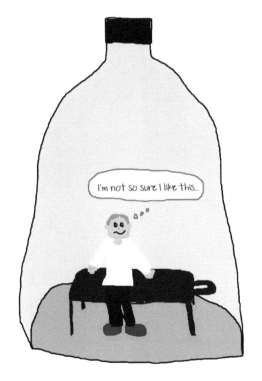

Okay, if you got to this page – you get the "bonus points" I guess. You probably have DiGize and Helichrysum – and are waiting to hear what they are good for...

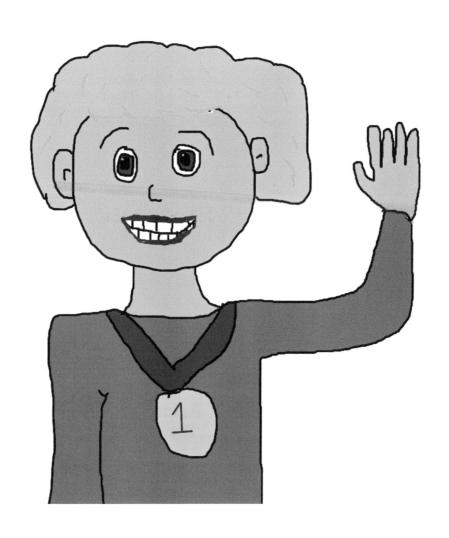

Helichrysum Essential Oil is the most wonderful, amazing, perfect oil on earth! It can stop bleeding, help blood clots and bruises go away faster, and my mom says it even helps with a HEART ATTACK!

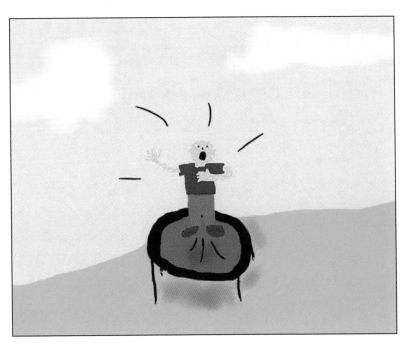

Sometimes we worry about grandpa or grandma when we ask them to skateboard or jump on the trampoline with us. So it is REALLY good to know about the heart attack thing!

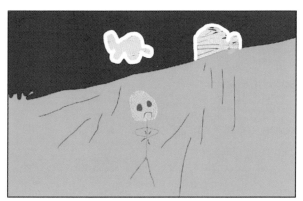

DiGize Essential Oil Blend is made for all sorts of things that might go wrong in your guts. Puking (mom said say vomiting), throwing up (vomiting), spewing (vomiting), tossing your cookies (vomiting gluten free cookies), up-chucking (vomiting), hurling (vomiting)...

OOPS, mom is coming...

It is also good for the squirts (yah, yah - I know - Diarrhea), car-sickness, nausea (almost vomiting).

We usually stick this oil in our belly button or on the bottom of our feet. It doesn't taste too great, but in a pinch, we have taken a few drops in an empty gelatin capsule.

It's good to know that if you think you have food poisoning or you need to vomit... DiGize can help you do that, too. Don't worry – it won't make you blow chunks if you don't need to...

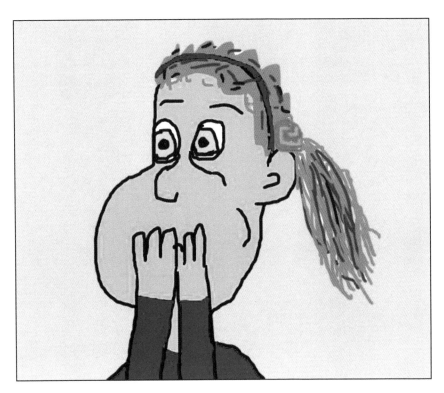

But in the words of one of our favorite green cartoon characters, sometimes things are "better out than in!"

We hope you have enjoyed our book! We really had a lot of fun writing it (and illustrating it!)

We think essential oils are pretty cool - and most people think so too after they get to use them.

If you want to know more about essential oils, order books, or get your own essential oils - you can visit my mom's websites:

www.OilyVet.com   or
                www.AnimalDeskReference.com

She's got WAY too much information on there... But, I guess it is kind of neat anyway.

19168213R00031

Made in the USA
Charleston, SC
09 May 2013